AF416651

Dedication Page

This book is a dedication to those who have endured the heartache and
of losing a loved one too soon. It is for the families who have bravely faced
grief and sorrow that comes with such a loss. I dedicate this work to my
family, who lost a bright light in our lives, and to all those who
experienced similar tragedies. The story that follows is a testament to
resilience of the human spirit and the power of love and support in the fa
adversity. It is a reminder that even in the darkest of times, there is alway
potential for growth, healing, and a path forward. This is for those who
walked through the valley of shadows and emerged with a newf
appreciation for life and all its fragility. As you read this, know that you ar
alone in your struggles. May these words bring comfort, hope, and
knowledge that even in the face of immense loss, there is always
possibility of finding peace and solace.

Preface: This book is to help the reader understand and learn w[...] improve their personal and physical life by eating healthy, exercis[...] mindset.

The book you hold in your hands is a powerful tool for transformation. It is a guide to help you become the best version of yourself, and to live a life of vitality, health, and happiness. Through a combination of healthy eating, exercise, meditation and a positive mindset, you will gain an understanding of how to improve your overall well-being. The journey to self-improvement and a life of wellness can be challenging, but with this book as your companion, you will navigate a path to success. This guide will empower you to take control of your physical and mental health, and in doing so, you will discover a happier and more fulfilling life.

It is an honest and practical road map to help you achieve your goals and aspirations, with a focus on simple, effective strategies. By embracing the teachings within these pages, you will gain a deeper understanding of the connection between your mind and body, and how to harness their power to create a better you. This book is an invitation to explore and embrace a healthier, more balanced lifestyle. It encourages you to take a step back, evaluate your current state, and make positive changes to enhance your overall well-being. Whether you seek to improve your physical health, gain mental clarity, or simply find a calmer and more positive mindset, this guide will be your constant companion, providing the tools and motivation to succeed.

As you turn each page, you will uncover a wealth of knowledge and practical advice. You will learn how to nourish your body with nutritious foods, move with intention and purpose through exercise, and calm your mind through meditation and a positive mindset practice. Each chapter builds upon the last, creating a comprehensive and holistic approach to your transformation.

Introduction:

Those of us in our 50's & 60's must change our mindset!

There are things that we can do to rewire our minds. We as men in our 50
60's must acknowledge that our minds are powerful tools that can e
empower or hinder us. The first step is to recognize that change is pos
and that we have the consciousness to rewire our thinking. It's time to let g
outdated mindsets and embrace a new way of thinking that will empower u
live more fulfilling and meaningful lives. There are several strategies we
employ to reshape our mindset. Firstly, we must challenge negative self
and replace it with positive, empowering affirmations. We should also surro
ourselves with like-minded individuals who encourage and support our gro
Seeking out new experiences and stepping out of our comfort zones can
us develop a more growth-oriented mindset. Additionally, we can u
visualization techniques to imagine ourselves successfully adopting a new
of thinking. By seeing ourselves as capable and adaptable, we can beg
embody these qualities in our daily lives. It's important to remember
changing our mindset is a journey, and progress may not always be li
However, with persistence and dedication, we can reshape our thinking
unlock a world of new possibilities.

Chapter 1 : The Problem Explained

As we age, many older men have the problem of unhealthy and negative habits. We wake up each morning and think about how we feel, how we are overweight and our muscles ache, but we don't have the motivation or mindset to make a change. As we enter our wiser years, some of us make life choices that are not so—very wise. Therefore, a unique set of challenges presents itself. Many of us find ourselves battling against this tide of unhealthy and negative habits that have taken root in our lives.

Each morning, we are faced with the stark reality of our physical condition; the extra weight that seems to have crept up unnoticed, or just the lack of concern and motivation to address our failing condition. It is a cycle that many of my peers find themselves trapped. We wake up, and the first thought that enters our mind is often a critical assessment of our physical state. We feel sluggish, our bodies seem to have betrayed us, and the idea of change seems daunting, if not impossible. The issue is not just the physical manifestation of our unhealthy habits, but the mindset that accompanies it. **WE ARE WHAT WE THINK!**

It is a vicious cycle; we feel unhealthy, so we lack the motivation to make positive changes, and this lack of motivation leads to further physical and mental stagnation. It becomes a downward spiral that many of us struggle to escape. The very idea of change seems like an insurmountable task, so we remain unmotivated with a negative mindset, trapped in a body and mentality that continues to fuel our unhappiness, we tell ourselves; I need to start eating healthier, or I have got to start working out and exercising, but life seems to get busier and busier and you continue to live in an unhealthy lifestyle. This is a problem that plagues men of our age but it even starts with some in their earlier years, it is a problem in our current society that needs addressing and therefore why I felt so compelled to write this book.

We find ourselves at a crossroads, knowing that something needs to change, yet we procrastinate to make that change. It is a mental and physical battle, and one that requires a shift in mindset and a re-evaluation of our habits. It is only then that we can hope to break free from this cycle and embrace a healthier, more positive future. We know the routine all too well: the groggy awakening, the sluggish trudge to the bathroom, the dull gaze at our reflection. We see the evidence of our bad habits etched on our faces and our bodies. The weight of our unhealthy choices bears down on us, yet we remain stagnant, trapped in a cycle of negative thinking and inaction.

What if today was different? What if, instead of succumbing to the familiar path of self-criticism and apathy, we chose to embrace a new mindset? A mindset of possibility, where we recognize our potential to forge a healthier, happier path. It starts with a simple decision, to prioritize our well-being and take small, manageable steps towards positive change. Instead of dwelling on our flaws, we focus on our strengths and use them as a foundation for growth. We set realistic goals, take joy in the process, and celebrate each small victory along the way. It's time to rewrite our story, to embrace the power of positive habits, and to create a future where we are not just surviving, but thriving. With positive affirmation you demand change, and tell yourself today will be the day! I now break free from my stagnant cycle, I am done with the unhealthy choices, it's time to develop a positive mindset and make healthy choices for my longevity and future. Below are ten steps with positive affirmations to start your journey, and as you progress you will achieve more power and confidence in your routine.

Positive Affirmations!

1. Start with a simple routine: waking up with purpose. No more grogginess, I will not fall into the trap of negative thinking, A quick energizing routine will be my morning ritual: a splash of cold water on my face, or a brisk shower, some light stretching, and a positive affirmation to set the tone.

2. Focus on nutrition. Out with the junk, in with the wholesome. My diet is my medicine. I am fueling my body with nutritious foods that make me feel energized and strong. I take joy in discovering new, healthy recipes and celebrating the flavors that nourish me.

3. Movement is motivation. Incorporate gentle exercises like walking and/or swimming into a daily routine, embracing the endorphin rush that follows.

4. Prioritize rest and recovery. Adequate sleep and relaxation techniques are my tools to recharge, ensuring I am refreshed and ready for each new day. Meditation is my ally, helping me stay focused and calm

5. I embrace self-care rituals. Taking care of personal hygiene and appearance boosts my confidence and self-esteem. A well-groomed man is a confident man, look into your mirror and state positive affirmations to yourself, (we are what we think)!

6. Set realistic goals and celebrate achievements. Small, manageable steps are my current strategy, ensuring I stay motivated and proud of my progress. Rewarding myself for each small victory keeps me driven and excited.

7. Surround yourself with positivity, inspiring books, uplifting music, and encouraging company are great support systems. Keep your mindset focused and optimistic.

8. Practice gratitude each day and reflect on the things for which to be thankful. Appreciate the little blessings and keep a positive outlook. Journal every morning and state your goals and achievements.

9. Take up a new hobby that is creative, that engages your mind and brings you joy. Try something that allows you to express yourself and feel a sense of fulfillment.

10. Most importantly, be kind to yourself. Self-love and self-acceptance are my foundation. I embrace my flaws and use them as motivation to improve and never dwell on my shortcomings. **I am empowered with a positive mindset and healthy choices to get back to where I desire to be.**

Chapter 2: The Evolution of Strength

As I delved deeper into the significance of healthy habits, I realized that it isn't just about physical appearance or even overall health. It is about empowerment and the ability to take on the world as a strong, confident man. This chapter, "The Evolution Of Strength" becomes the manifesto for men everywhere to take control of their lives and embrace a journey of transformation. The lack of attention to healthy eating and physical activity has led many down a dangerous path. Men are becoming softer, both physically and mentally, and it is impacting every aspect of our lives. From the boardroom to the bedroom, a lack of strength and stamina is evident, and it is time to address the root cause. It is time for men to reclaim their power and potential. By embracing a lifestyle of healthy eating and regular exercise, we can become the best version of ourselves. This isn't just about aesthetics or vanity; it is about building a strong foundation for a fulfilling life.

Physical strength translates into mental fortitude and soon men will be able to defend, support, and protect not just ourselves but also those around us. This journey isn't just about lifting weights and counting calories. It is a mental exercise, a re-evaluation of priorities, and a re-ignition of passion. Men will learn to channel their inner warrior, embrace challenges and overcome obstacles.

With each victory, big or small, we will feel a sense of accomplishment and a boost in confidence. But it's not just the individual who will benefit. Strong, healthy men contribute to strong, healthy communities. We become role models for the next generation, teaching them the value of self-care and personal development. It becomes a cycle of positive influence, with each man inspiring those around him to rise to their full potential. This chapter is a call to action, a rallying cry for men to embrace their true strength and forge a brighter future. We are energy and power!

Now onto our diets and how it affects our lives. We are not meant to eat three times a day and the food today in western culture has too many dangerous preservatives and additives for our bodies to consume. As a society, we have become accustomed to a lifestyle that is detrimental to our health. The issue lies in our modern eating habits and a lack of emphasis on physical education, resulting in a generation of individuals struggling with poor eating habits, weight issues, and chronic illnesses. It is time to recognize that we are energy beings and our current eating patterns, with three structured meals a day, may not align with our natural energetic needs. The food industry, unfortunately, does not help our cause with its rampant use of harmful preservatives.

To counter these issues, various diets have emerged, each with their own philosophy and approach to healthy eating. From the restrictive nature of calorie-counting diets to the liberating but challenging ketogenic diet, there are a wide range of options to choose from. Some advocate for a plant-based lifestyle, promoting the health benefits of a vegan or vegetarian diet, while others, like the paleo diet, encourage a return to our ancestral eating habits, focusing on whole, unprocessed foods. Intermittent fasting has also gained popularity, emphasizing when we eat as well as what we eat, allows flexibility in food choices within a designated eating window. With so many options available, it can be overwhelming to decide which path to take. Each diet has its own community of passionate advocates, swearing by its life-changing effects. But it is important to remember that there is no one-size-fits-all approach. As individuals, we must explore these options, educate ourselves, and make informed decisions about our health and dietary choices. It is a journey of self-discovery, and the first step is recognizing the need for change. The healthiest diet consists of natural meats and uncontaminated vegetables.

The importance of our bodies, our energy and mindset are vital for how we can be more aware of our sub-conscience and our inner energy. We as all creations are made up of energy. We are energy beings, a part of the vibrant tapestry of creation and it's time we started treating our bodies as the temples of energy they are. Our modern eating habits with, their structured meals and processed foods, have veered us off course from our natural energetic needs. It is no wonder so many of us struggle with our weight and health. But there is hope! A variety of diets have emerged, each offering a unique path to rediscovering our energetic balance. From calorie-counting to keto, plant-based to paleo, we now have a plethora of options to explore and educate ourselves. It can be daunting to navigate the passionate advocates of each diet, all claiming life-changing results. But remember, we are all unique energy systems, and what works for one may not work for another. It's a journey of self-discovery, an exploration of what fuels our individual fires. The first step is recognizing the need for change and understanding that we are not bound by the traditional three-meals-a-day structure. Our bodies, our energy, our needs are dynamic and ever-changing. Let's embrace the sun, the earth, and the natural, unadulterated foods they provide. Let's tap into our inner energy, listen to our bodies, and make conscious choices about what we fuel ourselves with. It's an exciting adventure, and I believe we can all find our path to energetic harmony and optimal health. The power is within us, and with each step, we become more attuned to our true nature.

Chapter 3: The Power of a Positive Mindset.

Society has conditioned us to be docile. We are often told what to think, how to act, and what to strive for. It's as if we are on autopilot, going through the motions without truly questioning or challenging our thoughts and actions. But we have the power to break free from this conditioning and reshape our mindset. It starts with recognizing the influence of our thoughts and the energy we put out into the world. A positive mindset is a powerful tool, and it begins with self-awareness. I had to teach myself to pay attention to my thoughts and the underlying beliefs that shape them. Are my thoughts serving me? Am I being too critical or pessimistic? By actively choosing positive thoughts and affirmations, I can shift my mindset and, consequently, my outlook on life. This is not to say that I ignore negative thoughts or suppress them. Instead, I acknowledge their presence without judgment and then gently guide my focus back to the positive. Meditation has become a vital practice in this journey. Each morning, I take a moment to sit in silence and observe my thoughts. I notice the worries, the to-do lists, and the external noise trying to invade my mind. But, with each breath, I let them go and return to the present moment. This practice has taught me to recognize the power of my thoughts and, more importantly, that I have the power to choose which thoughts to entertain.

Over time, meditation has helped me cultivate a sense of calm and clarity, allowing me to approach each day with a positive mindset and renewed energy. Maintaining a routine has also been essential. I start my days with meditation, followed by a gratitude practice and some light journaling. Throughout the day, set small, achievable goals and celebrate each victory. Before bed, reflect on the day's accomplishments and the lessons learned. This routine has helped me stay grounded and focused, ensuring that I begin and end each day with a positive mindset. It has become a cycle of self-improvement and personal growth, and I am excited to see the person I become as I continue this journey of self-discovery and positive thinking. I am under no illusion that this is an easy journey, and I know that old habits and negative thought patterns may try to resurface. But, with each challenge, I am committed to reminding myself of the power I hold within me – the power of a positive mindset.

Chapter 4: Strategies to change mindset.

I want to share with you some practical techniques that can help shift your mindset and outlook on life. These are strategies that I have personally used and refined over the years, and I truly believe they can help you create a more positive and hopeful mindset. One of the most powerful tools I've discovered is the practice of gratitude. Each day, take a moment to reflect on the things you are thankful for. It could be as simple as the warm sun on your face or the sound of your child's laughter. By actively practicing gratitude, you train your brain to seek out the positive aspects of your life, no matter how big or small. This simple exercise has the power to shift your focus and create a more optimistic outlook. Another strategy I've found effective is to challenge negative self-talk. We all have an inner critic, but it's important to recognize when this voice becomes overly critical or pessimistic. When you notice negative self-talk, pause and ask yourself if you would say those same things to a friend. More often than not, the answer is no. Treat yourself with the same kindness and compassion you would show to others. Replace those negative thoughts with more positive, realistic statements. For example, instead of thinking, "I always mess everything up," try, "I didn't achieve the outcome I wanted this time, but I can learn from this and do better next time.

Visualization is another powerful technique for mindset change. Spend time each day visualizing your goals and dreams as if they have already come true. Create a mental image of your future success, and really engage your senses in this vision. See the details, hear the sounds, and feel the emotions associated with your accomplishment. This practice helps to reinforce a positive mindset and keeps you focused on your aspirations. It also serves as a daily reminder that your goals are achievable and worth pursuing.

Becoming a better version of yourself is the goal, and it starts with your physical and mental health. You want to be healthier, more positive, and have more energy? Devise a plan with actionable steps to achieve these goals and become the man you want to be. First, assess your eating habits. Eliminate processed foods and incorporate more whole, natural foods into your diet. Start meal prepping to ensure you always have nutritious options available. You can also begin taking daily multivitamins to ensure your body is getting all the nutrients it needs.

Knowing that exercise is crucial for both physical and mental health, makes it a non-negotiable part of your routine. Commit to working out a minimum of three times a week. I have found a home gym to work out to reach my fitness goals. It motivates me to stay on track and pushes me to new fitness heights. Meditate and make it your tool to cultivate a positive mindset. Each morning, dedicate 15 minutes to quiet reflection, focusing on your breath and setting an intention for the day. This practice helps you start each day with a sense of calm and purpose. To further surround yourself with positivity, begin writing in a gratitude journal each morning, reflecting on the good things you plan during the day and expressing gratitude for what you received the day prior. You will start to understand the importance of routines and schedules and in maintaining a healthy lifestyle.

Structure your days to include time for self-care, work, and social activities. Make sure to get enough sleep each night, as it is crucial for your energy levels and overall health. Set boundaries to ensure you are not taking on more than you could handle, learning to say no when necessary to avoid overwhelming yourself. Lastly, Distanced yourself from negative influences. Surround yourself with like-minded, positive people who support your journey and uplift you. Avoid situations that bring unnecessary stress or negativity into your life, choose instead to focus on the good and maintain a sense of peace and optimism. These steps will help transform your life, and feel like a new man, you will have more energy, a positive outlook, and control over your life.

Chapter 6: Embracing Positive Thinking

In my journey towards self-improvement, I discovered the power of positive thinking. It's incredible how much of an impact our thoughts can have on our overall well-being and the direction of our lives. To guide me on this path, I turned to books like "What You Say to Yourself" and "As a Man Thinketh." These books emphasize the importance of positive affirmations and the power of our thoughts in shaping our reality. By adopting a positive mindset, I believe I attract positive outcomes and improve my overall happiness and satisfaction with life. I begin each day with a positive affirmation, repeating to myself, "I am strong, I am powerful, I am young, I will live to be 120, I am worthy, I am capable, " This simple yet powerful phrase boosted my confidence and set a positive tone for the day. I want to emphasize again how very important this part of your routine is for your success,

Write down three things you are thankful for each morning in your gratitude journal. This practice helps you focus on the positive aspects of your life, no matter how small, and cultivates a sense of appreciation and contentment. To stay motivated and inspired, utilize planners and templates. Trello is your trusted companion, it can assist you in organizing your thoughts, setting goals, and create actionable plans. Design a board specifically for your self-improvement journey, with columns for short-term and long-term goals, with cards detailing the steps needed to take to achieve them. Each card is called a rock, they are like a small, achievable milestones, and moving them across the board gives you a sense of progress and accomplishment. Additionally, discover the power of worksheets. You can find a fantastic resource online—a comprehensive worksheet packet designed to guide individuals towards a healthier and more positive mindset. It includes sections for self-reflection, goal setting, and creating actionable plans. The worksheets may help you delve deeper into your thoughts and emotions, uncovering any negative thought patterns and replacing them with positive, empowering beliefs.

Chapter 7: Developed Personalized Action Plan.

I want to share the steps I took on my road to living a Positive healthy a life, so you will know, it actually works when they are applied. It is si what I recommended for you so you may think I am being redundan

Personal Journey to Positive Transformation I knew it was time for a cha
and that meant taking control and developing an action plan for my life.
chapter marks the beginning of my journey towards a positive mindset
improved health, with specific, manageable goals and a personalized stra
First, I needed to define my goals and ensure they were realistic
achievable. So, I started with a broad overview, setting a primary go
improving my overall health and well-being. This included physical he
mental and emotional resilience, and a more positive outlook on life. To n
this goal manageable, I broke it down into smaller, specific targets: impro
my diet and sleep habits, incorporating regular exercise, developir
mindfulness practice, and setting aside free time for hobbies and outings.
these goals in mind, I structured my days to include time for self-care
personal development. Each morning, I dedicated 15 minutes to planning
day and visualizing my success. I also incorporated a nightly review to re
on my progress and adjust my plan as needed. This daily ritual helped me
focused and accountable. Time management was key to my succe
scheduled my days to ensure I had time for my health and self-improver
goals. I woke up earlier to fit in a morning workout and meditation session,
I prepared healthy meals in advance to save time and make nutritious chc
easier. I also scheduled 'me time' for reading, hobbies, and social activ
ensuring a balanced approach to self-care. To stay motivated, I trackec
progress and celebrated small wins. I kept a journal to record
achievements and reflect on how far I'd come. I also treated myself to s
rewards along the way, like a new book or a day trip on my Harle
acknowledge my hard work and keep me driven. This journey wasn't wit
its challenges, but my determination to stay on course and my belief
brighter future kept me going. With each step, I felt stronger and r
capable, and the positive changes in my life fueled my continued dedicatic
my action plan. This chapter serves as a template for others to create
own personalized journeys towards a brighter, healthier future. It is a remi
that with goal setting, time management, and a belief in oneself, pos
transformation is achievable and sustainable.

When you make the decision to change your mentality and your
mindset, you can do amazing things, someone who isn't at this level
of peace and energy will probably disagree, but once they take the
journey, they will change their mind. This is a way of life and a new
beginning for men that are struggling personally , physically and
even professionally in their lives. This is a transformational journey
and one you will always appreciate.

Chapter 8: Overcoming Obstacles

There will be obstacles and bumps in the road, we must stay vigilant in our quest to become who we are designed to be. The path to self-discovery and fulfillment is rarely smooth. It is often filled with challenges and obstacles that test our resolve and character. But it is in these moments of adversity that we have the opportunity to grow and showcase our resilience. you will face many hurdles in your journey and rest assured, I know there will be more ahead. Yet, you must remain steadfast in your quest to become the person you are designed to be.

Vigilance and perseverance are your allies in this endeavor. You will understand that the road to success is paved with determination and hard work. One of the biggest challenges you'll encounter is a period of self-doubt and imposter syndrome; questioning your abilities and whether you are truly on the right path. It may feel like walking through a dense fog, unsure of your next step and uncertain of your direction, your bad habits will change after 20 days of consistency, so refuse to let these doubts consume you. Seek guidance from mentors and surround yourself with a supportive network who lifts you up and reminds you of your strengths and how important this journey is. Learn to silence the inner critic and replace self-doubt with self-belief, Other obstacles will come in the form of unexpected change, handle these obstacles and empower yourself. Life sometimes throws curveballs, as we are forced to adapt and navigate uncharted territories on a path of self-improvement.

 For me, it was a sudden shift in my personal life that left me feeling lost and uncertain. However, I embraced my resilience and adaptability. I realized that change could bring new opportunities and a fresh perspective. I learned to embrace the unknown and trust in my ability to navigate any situation. I also encountered challenges in the form of setbacks and failures. There were times when I didn't achieve my goals, despite my best efforts. But I refused to let these moments define me. Instead, I chose to view them as lessons and steppingstones to success. I analyzed my mistakes, learned from them, and used them as fuel to propel me forward, understanding that growth often comes from our lowest moments, and it is in our power to rise again stronger and wiser. Overcoming these obstacles has made me realize that the journey to self-improvement and success is not linear. It is filled with twists and turns, highs and lows. But by staying vigilant and adaptable, we can navigate any challenge that comes our way. I continue my journey, embracing the bumps in the road, knowing that they are all part of my success.

Chapter 9: Building Habits

We must be consistent in our journey, no one will do it for us and we, as men, should always be the greatest strength of our families. The path to success is paved with consistency and perseverance. As men, we bear the responsibility of being the bedrock of our families, and this demands a steadfast commitment to our goals and an unwavering dedication to self-improvement. Understanding that our actions have a profound impact on those around us, especially our loved ones, is crucial. Building new habits and cultivating a disciplined mindset are essential to this endeavor. It is imperative that we recognize the significance of consistency and the power it holds to transform our lives. By establishing a routine and sticking to it, we forge a path toward our desired future, step by step.

Habit tracking has emerged as a potent tool in this regard. Numerous techniques and tools are available to assist individuals in holding themselves accountable and monitoring their progress. One effective method is the use of habit-tracking applications. These apps serve as digital companions, providing structure and motivation. They allow users to set daily goals, receive reminders, and track their progress over time. Visual representations of progress, such as charts and graphs, offer a tangible sense of accomplishment and encourage continued dedication. However, it is worth noting that technology is not always necessary for habit formation. Some individuals find the act of writing by hand to be a meditative practice that enhances their commitment to their goals. The physical act of crossing off tasks or filling in a calendar can be immensely satisfying and serve as a powerful motivator. For those seeking a more creative approach, vision boards can be a powerful tool. This involves curating a collage of images, quotes, and reminders that represent one's goals and desired habits. Placed in a visible location, it serves as a constant reminder of one's aspirations, inspiring and motivating one to stay on course. The key to success lies in finding an approach that resonates personally and then committing to it fully. Consistency is the cornerstone of habit formation, and by embracing this mindset, we set ourselves on the path to achieving our aspirations and becoming the bedrock of support and inspiration for those we hold dear.

Habits are activities with repetitiveness, they can be changed by doing different things in a repetitive action, 20 days and you can change any habit. Consistency is the key, positive mindset and affirmations are the answer, regaining your Alpha is your resolution.

Chapter 10: Staying Motivated

We all get busy and side tracked from time to time, life can hit us with unexpected and negative issues. So now we will cover ways to stay motivated in tough times. Life has a tendency to throw curveballs our way when we least expect it. Staying motivated during these challenging periods is essential for personal growth and resilience. Here are some strategies to help you navigate through life's obstacles and maintain a positive mindset. First and foremost, it's crucial to accept that setbacks and challenges are an inevitable part of life. Instead of resisting or fighting against them, embrace them as opportunities for growth and self-improvement. This shift in perspective can help you stay motivated and resilient. For example, if you lose your job unexpectedly, try to view it as a chance to explore a new career path or develop your skills further. Setting clear and defined goals can also help you stay motivated during tough times. Break down your goals into smaller, achievable tasks, and celebrate each milestone you reach.

This sense of accomplishment will motivate you to keep going and provide a feeling of progress, even during challenging periods. For instance, if your goal is to run a marathon, set smaller targets, such as increasing your running distance by a certain amount each week, and reward yourself when you achieve these milestones. Surrounding yourself with a supportive network is another crucial aspect of staying motivated. Lean on your friends, family, or a support group during tough times. Their encouragement and belief in you can help lift your spirits and remind you of your strengths. Additionally, seek out mentors or individuals who have overcome similar challenges, as they can provide valuable guidance and inspiration. Self-care is also essential for maintaining motivation. Take care of your physical and mental health, especially during stressful periods. Engage in activities that help you relax and recharge, such as meditation, yoga, or spending time in nature. Prioritizing self-care will help you stay energized and focused, making it easier to tackle challenges head-on. For example, if you're feeling overwhelmed, take a break and go for a walk in a park to clear your mind and rejuvenate yourself. Lastly, stay focused on the present moment and take things one step at a time.

Instead of getting overwhelmed by the bigger picture, break down your tasks or goals into manageable chunks. Focus on what you can control and take small, consistent actions toward your goals. This will help you build momentum and maintain motivation, even during the most challenging times. Remember, staying motivated is a personal journey, and you might need to adapt these strategies to fit your unique situation. Be kind to yourself, stay resilient, and always look for the learning opportunities that life's challenges present.

I am offering a mentorship, coaching sessions and will be opening a chat group for men who wish to participate or want to be involved with like-minded men who are transforming their lives, you can find my contact info on the copyright section of this book. We are never done becoming a better man—better versions of ourselves.

Conclusion

The book has been an eye-opening journey, offering a wealth of insights and practical strategies for personal growth and development. As I reflect on the key messages, I am reminded of the power of self-belief and the importance of taking proactive steps towards our goals. Throughout these pages, we have explored the intricacies of personal transformation, uncovering the steps to unlock our true potential. We have discovered the power of mindset, the necessity of self-care, and the impact of our habits on our overall success. By providing actionable advice and real-world examples, this book has equipped us with the tools to create positive change in our lives. One of the standout messages for me is the emphasis on taking responsibility for our own growth. The book encourages us to embrace a growth mindset, understanding that challenges and setbacks are opportunities for development rather than obstacles to fear. By adopting this mindset, we can approach life with a sense of resilience and adaptability, confident in our ability to learn and evolve. Another key takeaway is the importance of self-care. Taking time to nurture our physical, mental, and emotional well-being is not a luxury but a necessity. The book highlights the impact of stress and burnout, offering strategies to manage our energy and maintain a healthy work-life balance. By prioritizing self-care, we can show up as our best selves in all areas of life.

Furthermore, the book delves into the science of habit formation, providing a framework for building positive habits and breaking free from negative ones. By understanding the habit loop and utilizing strategies such as cue replacement and reward substitution, we can design our daily routines to support our goals and aspirations. As I reflect on my journey through these pages, I am filled with a sense of empowerment and excitement for the future. The book has not only provided theoretical knowledge but also practical steps to implement immediately. I hope you are motivated to apply the lessons learned, such as setting meaningful goals, creating a positive environment, and building a supportive community around yourself. Please recognize that growth is an ongoing process, and true transformation takes time and dedication. As you continue on your path, re-visit key chapters and reflect on the exercises to reinforce your learning. Additionally, seek out supplementary resources, such as podcasts, online courses, and mentorship programs, to further enhance understanding and stay motivated.

Finally, I encourage all readers to embrace the lessons within these pa take action. Personal growth is an individual journey, and by apply strategies outlined, we can each create a life of fulfillment and purpo this book be a catalyst for positive change, inspiring us to unlock potential and live the lives we desire. As I conclude, I am reminded of by author and philosopher Lao Tzu, "A journey of a thousand miles with a single step." May this book be that first step towards a brigh more fulfilling future for us all. Let's embark on this journey t embracing the power of personal growth and transformation.

Acknowledgements

I would like to thank my son for giving me the inspiration to become a better man, for your invaluable support and My Amazing wife and best friend, Amy, for your contributions to this book. Your encouragement and assistance have been instrumental in the completion of this work. I LOVE YOU!

Appendices

References:

Self improvement books

> Positive thinking affirmations
> The power of consistency
> As a man thinketh
> Scientific healing affirmations
> Atomic habits
> Rich Dad poor dad

About the Author

I, Patrick Gardner, came into this world on July 25, 1964, in Dallas, Texas. But my story truly began when my family moved to Oklahoma, where I spent my formative years. As the third son, I had a brother, a sister, and several half-siblings, which made for a lively household. I was a shy boy, but I found an outlet for my energy in wrestling, a sport that would teach me discipline and give me an early taste of what it meant to be physically and mentally strong. My journey into manhood continued when I joined the military, serving my country with pride. The experiences I had and the comrades I made during this time shaped me into the leader I am today. After my military career, I found myself drawn to the world of construction, starting as a worker but soon rising through the ranks to become a manager. It was a natural progression, as I had always possessed a take charge mindset that seemed to drive me towards leadership roles. Now, I find myself embarking on a new venture: writing my first book. It is a project born out of a desire to help men who, like me, have faced challenges and struggled to maintain a positive mindset and their place as leaders in their own lives. It is a guide, a companion, and a testament to the will of the masculine spirit.